POWER ISO-BOW POWER PUMP Method

POWER ISO-BOW
POWER PUMP

Method

The Best Isotonic/Isometric programs that build muscle mass, increase power, and sculpt your best body Today!

BECOME A ISO-BOW MAN!

The Power Iso-Bow Power Pump Method was written to help you get closer to your physical potential when it comes to real muscle sculpting strengthening exercises. The exercises and routines in this book are quite demanding, so consult your physician and have a physical exam taken prior to the start of this exercise program. Proceed with the suggested exercises and information at your own risk. The Publishers and author shall not be liable or responsible for any loss, injury, or damage allegedly arising from the information or suggestions in this book.

Power Iso-Bow Power Pump Method
muscle-building Course

By

Birch Tree Publishing
Published by Birch Tree Publishing

Power Iso-Bow Power Pump Method
Published in 2020, All rights reserved,
No part of this book may be reproduced, scanned,
or distributed in any printed or electronic form without permission.

Birch Tree Publishing

Dedication

For Mr. Popeye Spinach John Hughes, The Iso-Bow **POWER PUMP METHOD**

Contents

Introduction: BY JOHN HUGHES   **PG 7**

Chapter 1: MUSCLE FIBER ANALYSIS **RECAP**   **PG 11**

Chapter 2: BUILD A POWERFUL CHEST   **PG 14**

Chapter 3: DEVELOP POWERFUL SHOULDERS   **PG 17**

Chapter 4: DEVELOP A POWERFUL V-TAPER   **PG 22**

Chapter 5: DEVELOP POWERFUL BICEPS   **PG 28**

Chapter 6: DEVELOP POWERFUL TRICEPS   **PG 32**

Chapter 7: DEVELOP RIPPED FOREARMS   **PG 37**

Chapter 8: DEVELOP POWERFUL THIGHS   **PG 39**

Chapter 9: DEVELOP POWERFUL LOWER BACK   **PG 43**

Chapter 10: DEVELOP SHAPELY CALVES   **PG 46**

Chapter 11: DEVELOP RIPPED ABS   **PG 49**

Chapter 12: THE POWER PUMP STANDARD PROGRAM PHASE 1   **PG 55**

Chapter 13: THE POWER PUMP STANDARD PROGRAM PHASE 2   **PG 65**

Chapter 14: POWER PUMP FIBER FUSION   **PG 66**

Chapter 15: THE POWER PUMP POWER SURGE PHASE 1,2,3   **PG 78**

GET "ISO-BOW" STRONG

Introducing the worlds fastest physique enhancing series

Introduction by John Hughes

I have been involved with athletics all of my life, from college wrestling to World Championship Master's Wrestling in my 60s. Coupled with over 15 years of high school coaching, I have always strived for top physical performance in strength and flexibility for myself and the athletes I coached. I purchased my first Bullworker in the 1960s and was impressed with how quickly my body responded to Bullworker strength training. The portability of the product meant I never had to get rid of it due to space restraints and over the next 30 years, the ability to supplement any exercise routine with a quick Bullworker workout, always complimented my desired fitness goal.

In 1999, I became the North American distributor for Bullworker and began to work on design changes to make the product much more challenging, yet always maintaining the portability aspect of this time tested and proven fitness product. In recognizing the importance of cross-training principles for maximum fitness results, I designed additional products that kept with the Bullworker portability concept with each product able to be used either separately or combined for maximum fitness results in a complete cross-training program.

In 2010, I purchased most of the Global rights to Bullworker and have reintroduced Bullworker training principles that have been effective since 1962 and resulted in over 10 million units sold. Proven as the ultimate portable fitness products, Bullworker continues to deliver results to everyone, any age, wherever they exercise.

Now, I present the Iso-Bow Power Series. This book is about transforming your body, mind and spirit, which is what health, strength and physique enhancement is all about. I am really excited and positive to say that once you try the programs in this book, you will make some of the best gains you've ever made.

Join the men and women that are already using The Bullworker Power Series and programs with great success. **GET TRANSFORMED** today.

Keep pulling and pushing

Yours in Strength and Power

John Hughes

LET'S GO

LET'S GO

If you are reading this book, you already appreciate the importance of exercising for health, strength and wellbeing. The Power Iso-Bow Transformation Method will turn you into a powerful well built man. Being a great success at exercising means constant practice to transform yourself to become the best you can be.

When it comes to training-like most everything else in life-sometimes circumstances seem to get in the way from allowing you to exercise. Now, thanks to The Power Iso-Bow Method, you will always get a great workout-no matter where you are.

Resistance strength training with The Power Iso-Bow Method enhances:

1) Resistance strength training stimulates muscles to burn more calories than anything else. After your workout your metabolism is triggered for 40 hours after the session.
2) Your body will take on a different shape, and your clothes will fit far better.
3) Your flexibility will increase and resistance training will keep you young.
4) Your bones will become stronger. We lose bone mass as we get older, but resistance strength training increases bone density and add greater strength.
5) A stronger and healthy heart with enhanced blood flow.
6) Stress levels will be reduced due to exercise.
7) Resistance strength training also creates better sleeping patterns.
8) "No need to get depressed". Regular resistance training will ward off symptoms of depression.
9) Mental sharpness will be developed. This takes place due resistance training decreasing blood levels of homocysteine, the protein that's linked to developing Alzheimer's and dementia. Plus, resistance training enhances cognitive function. Workouts will improve memory and you will have longer attention spans.
10) Develop lazar-like focus.

The Training Series
that will create

a

Powerful
Iso-Bow Body

Chapter 1:
MUSCLE FIBER ANALYSIS (RECAP)

How Isotonics increases powerful muscles

Create the body of your dreams with Iso-Bow

01 MUSCLE FIBER ANALYSIS

In all truth, there are so many so-called theories floating around, it's hard to separate muscle-building fact from fiction. For many years, it was gospel that fast twitch 2Bs were best for muscle growth.

These were the supposedly **GET BIG** fibers. Truhfully, the true **KINGS** to muscle growth are the type 2As—the fibers that are fast-twitch, with an endurance element. This however, gives the trainee a double **BOOM** with a size and conditioning effect. Once done correctly.

Guess work does not exist within these pages. Our exercise Director Marlon Birch has taken all guess work out due to his muscle-building experience. Our rep range and methods stimulate and develop the important endurance fast twitch fibers that is important for enhancing muscle growth and increasing strength gains.

Our program stresses the muscles being worked to its maximum and not the tendons. Critical development from endurance-oriented fibers does not occur unless you keep tension time and the length of the set at 30 seconds and beyond.

2A fibers have both endurance and anaerobic capabilities, so to get the most growth, you need to tax both facets of the muscle for optimum size gains. So will a low rep range build any muscle at all? Low reps build muscle, but growth is slow and limited until the endurance-oriented capacities are taxed. This then stimulates the 2A fast-twitch fibers that promote muscle growth.

This is why the trainee needs to stay within the 20 rep range mark, this increases the load time placed on the fibers for serious growth and development to occur. 30 plus seconds will coax the size principal where low-threshold units are called first to fire, followed by the mediums, then the high threshold units. This is the best way to stimulate many fiber types to fire rapidly. However, the aerobic component of the fast-twitch fibers will be called into place promoting more muscle growth.

01 MUSCLE FIBER ANALYSIS

We design our programs to activate endurance fast twitch 2As, and extend the capacity in the ones that are firing rapidly. This however, makes the set 10 times more effective at promoting optimum muscle increase. Priming the nervous system and stimulating more blood blockage, which expands the internal structures of the muscle cell. So low reps do not tax the fast-twitch fibers enough to stimulate optimum muscle growth.

Chapter 2:

CHEST

BUILD A POWERFUL CHEST

BUILD A POWERFUL CHEST

02 BUILD A POWERFUL CHEST

The chest muscles allow you to push or move the arm forward or across
the body. These muscles are activated in any throwing or pushing motion.
Aesthetically, building a powerful chest is a sign of power in men.

However, the chest muscles are not used daily, so most times they are under
developed. So despite, the simplicity of how these muscles contract, they
can be trained in a number of various angles of push and pull, each offer its
own special muscle enhancing properties.

CHEST EXERCISES

02 BUILD A POWERFUL CHEST

INCLINE PUSHUPS

Place your hands on two chairs that are 15 inches high, the higher you go the greater pre-stretch there is. At the bottom position to enhance muscle-building stimuli, pause for 2 seconds before reversing the movement. This is an excellent warm up before your chest contraction exercises.

CHEST CONTRACTION

Cross arms as shown press the arms in opposite directions maintaining the tension. **(Isometric Contraction)** Now move your arm upwards and overhead, then reverse the motion maintaining strong tension. **DUAL ACTION**

Chapter 3:

SHOULDERS

DEVELOP POWERFUL SHOULDERS

DEVELOP POWERFUL SHOULDERS

03 DEVELOP POWERFUL SHOULDERS

The shoulder muscles are divided into three heads and are quite unique and move the arm in all directions. The front muscle raise the arm forward, the side muscles made up of a number of muscle bundles, and raises the arm out to the sides. The rear or posterior muscle, is designed to pull the arm backwards. Shoulder presses is a multi-muscle-use exercise, which is a compound exercise. This exercise recruits the front and side heads of the shoulders that tie in well with stimulating the upper and mid-back muscles as well giving the entire girdle complete development.

SHOULDER EXERCISES

03 DEVELOP POWERFUL SHOULDERS

Grasp the Iso-Bow in front of the body, as shown. Gradually raise the arm forward against the resistance of the other hand. **RESIST IN THE UP MOTION ONLY** This works the front part of the shoulder muscles.

SHOULDER EXERCISES

03 DEVELOP BARN DOOR SHOULDERS

LATERAL RAISES

Hold the Iso-Bow at waist, keep your elbows slightly bent, raise your arm as shown while resisting with the other arm. Perform all reps on one side first before switching arms. **RESIST IN ONE DIRECTION ONLY**

SHOULDER EXERCISES

03 DEVELOP POWERFUL SHOULDERS

ACROSS THE BODY PULLS

Place the Iso-Bow at chest height, keep your elbows slightly bent, pull the arm toward the right while resisting with the other arm. Pause and reverse the motion alternating sides. **DUAL ACTION RESIST IN BOTH DIRECTIONS**

Chapter 4:

UPPER BACK
DEVELOP A POWERFUL V-TAPER

DEVELOP A POWERFUL V-TAPER

04 DEVELOP A POWERFUL V-TAPER

The entire back is made up of many muscles overlapping each other. However, most trainees find the back quite difficult to fully develop. The reason? As the saying goes out of sight, out of mind. We cannot directly see the back muscles, plus we cannot see it flex like we would see the biceps.

We make training the entire back musculature much easier making developing the back obviously simple once you know what you are doing, you can bring these muscles up to speed. We are looking at the large Latissimus that covers the majority of the back. The trapezius is broken up into two sections.

UPPER BACK EXERCISES

04 DEVELOP A POWERFUL V-TAPER

DO NOT NEGLECT THE MID AND LOWER TRAPS

The upper traps and mid-back muscles. Plus, we have the teres major, which is strongly stimulated with unilateral work, which makes self resistance the ideal movement. The infraspinatus muscle is like a half circle on each side of the upper back and is a very important rotator cuff muscle.

This muscle stabilizes the shoulder and prevents dislocations. Even though this muscle is at the back, most traditional exercises do not fully target these muscles. However, with self resistance there are exercises that target this area for full development.

UPPER BACK EXERCISES

04 DEVELOP A POWERFUL V-TAPER

PULLDOWNS

Grasp the Iso-Bow as shown in the picture. Gradually pull the arm downwards while resisting with the bottom arm. **RESIST IN ONE DIRECTION ONLY**

UPPER BACK EXERCISES

04 DEVELOP A POWERFUL V-TAPER

UPPER BACK ROWS

Bring your arm across the body pre-stretching the mid-back, grasp the Iso-Bow as shown. Slowly pull the arm across the body toward the armpit against the resistance supplied by the other arm. Extend the arm back to the starting position. Repeat the movement, then switch arms. This adds thickens to the mid-back, lats, and biceps along with the rear part of the shoulders.
RESIST IN A DUAL MANNER

UPPER BACK EXERCISES

04 DEVELOP A POWERFUL V-TAPER

ADD POWER TO THE ROTATOR CUFF MUSCLES

Hold the Iso-Bow as shown. Pull the arms towards the middle of the exercise position, pause for 1 second, then proceed to the opposite side. **RESIST IN A DUAL MANNER**

Chapter 5:

BICEPS
DEVELOP POWERFUL BICEPS

DEVELOP POWERFUL BICEPS

05 DEVELOP POWERFUL BICEPS

The biceps muscle has two heads. A short head, which is on the inside of the arm, and a long head, which is on the outside. This is the part that people see first. The main roll of the biceps is to flex the forearm by bringing the hand towards the shoulder. In order to build powerful complete biceps, you need to learn that the biceps do not work by itself.

The brachialis, which is under the bicep when developed, gives the bicep a larger and fuller appearance. Performing curls place undesirable tension on the tendon near the elbow. In other words, the biceps is placed in a very vulnerable position. Always start all bicep exercises with a slight bend at the start and finish. Always maintain tension on the biceps and not the joint.

BICEPS

TRICEPS

BICEP EXERCISES

05 DEVELOP POWERFUL BICEPS

CONCENTRATION CURLS

As pictured, pull the right arm towards the face while resisting with the left hand. Now reverse the exercise by pushing the left arm down and resisting with the right. Complete your reps then switch arms and repeat movement. **DUAL ACTION**

BICEP EXERCISES

05 DEVELOP POWERFUL BICEPS

PALM UP CURLS

Pull the right arm upward towards the shoulder while resisting with the left hand. At the shoulder, reverse the exercise by pushing the left arm downwards, resisting with the right.

Chapter 6:

TRICEPS
DEVELOP POWERFUL TRICEPS

DEVELOP POWERFUL TRICEPS

06 DEVELOP POWERFUL TRICEPS

DEVELOP POWERFUL TRICEPS

The triceps has three heads: The lateral head, middle head and the long head. The role of the triceps is to straighten the arm. The triceps work in opposition to the biceps and brachialis muscles. The triceps has three heads this makes it much larger in mass than the biceps and the brachialis.

Unfortunately, most pay attention to the biceps, leaving the triceps under-developed. The lateral head, which is on the outside is what people see first. The triceps are easy to develop and we have made it easy for the trainee to achieve this.

TRICEP EXERCISES

06 DEVELOP POWERFUL TRICEPS

FORWARD EXTENSIONS

As shown above, press the right arm forward while resisting with the left hand. **Do not straighten the elbow.**
RESIST IN A DUAL MANNER

TRICEP EXERCISES

06 DEVELOP POWERFUL TRICEPS

OVERHEAD TRICEP EXTENSIONS

Place arms overhead, press the right arm upwards while resisting with the left arm. Use a light to moderate tension due to the tricep tendons being sensitive at that position. **Do not straighten the elbow. RESIST IN ONE DIRECTION ONLY**

TRICEP EXERCISES

06 DEVELOP POWERFUL TRICEPS

TRICEP PRESSDOWN

As pictured above, press the right hand downwards while resisting with the left arm. Repeat desired reps then switch arms. **RESIST IN ONE DIRECTION ONLY**

DEVELOP RIPPED FOREARMS

07 DEVELOP RIPPED FOREARMS

DEVELOP RIPPED FOREARMS

DEVELOP RIPPED FOREARMS

Forearm muscles are involved in every daily activity, just like the calves and abdominals. We use these muscles all the time, when we drive, write, type, hold a bag and even open a door.

Many of the muscles of the forearm deal with Muscle-multi-use. When you are moving the elbow by lowering and raising the forearm. Moving the wrist up and down by, plus raising and lowering the hand. All self resistance exercises stress the forearms to contract which will increase your grip strength.

FOREARM EXERCISES

07 DEVELOP RIPPED FOREARMS

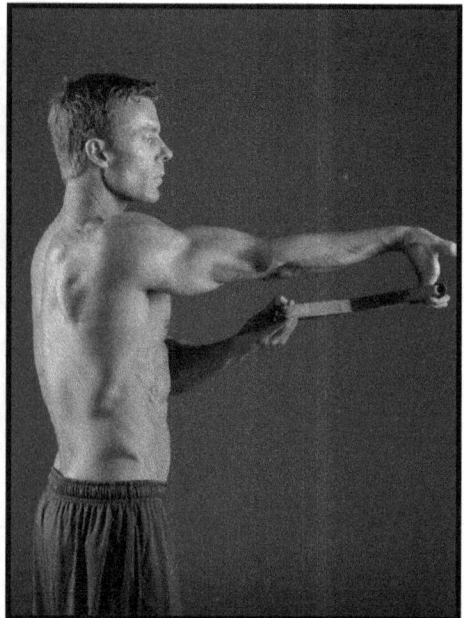

EXERCISE ONE   **EXERCISE TWO**

HAND/FOREARM EXERCISE

EXERCISE ONE: As pictured press the right hand forward until the fingers are pointed towards your feet. Return to position and repeat. **RESIST IN ONE DIRECTION**

EXERCISE TWO: Same as exercise one but, the hand is placed downwards.

Chapter 8:

THIGHS
DEVELOP POWERFUL THIGHS

DEVELOP POWERFUL TIRELESS THIGHS

08 DEVELOP POWERFUL TIRELESS THIGHS

DEVELOP POWERFUL THIGHS

The thigh muscles are basically made up of four main muscles: the vastus lateral muscle, this is located on the outside of the thighs. The vastus medial muscle, this is located on the inside of the thigh muscles towards the knee.

Better known as the tear drop because of its shape. The recus-femoris, which is located in the center of the muscles, and the vastus intermedius, this muscle is mostly covered by all the other muscles of the thighs. Our program will develop tireless thighs with a power pack punch.

LEG EXERCISES

08 DEVELOP POWERFUL TIRELESS THIGHS

LEG EXTENSIONS

While seated on a chair, box or stool, place the legs as shown in the picture. Now extend the left leg outwards resisting with the right. At the top pause for 2 seconds, then reverse the movement by pulling down with the right while resisting with the left. **DO NOT STRAIGHTEN THE KNEE. RESIST IN A DUAL MANNER**

LEG EXERCISES

08 DEVELOP POWERFUL TIRELESS THIGHS

LEG PRESS

As shown, pull the right leg towards the chest, powerfully resisting with the left leg. At the finished position, press the left foot forward resisting with the right. **PERFORM IN A DUAL MANNER**

Chapter 9:

LOWER BACK
DEVELOP POWERFUL LOWER-BACK MUSCLES

DEVELOP POWERFUL LOWER BACK MUSCLES

09 DEVELOP POWERFUL LOWER-BACK MUSCLES

POWERFUL LOWER BACK MUSCLES

Develop Powerful Lower back muscles
The lower back muscles support the lower part of the spine.
When these muscles are well developed it builds a brace protecting the spine.

Apart from that the lower back muscles are responsible for bringing the body upright from a leaning forward position. Not only will the lower back be involved, but the glutes and hamstrings come into play.

LOWER BACK EXERCISES

09 DEVELOP POWERFUL LOWER BACK

LOWER BACK EXTENSION

As shown above, this is the finished position. Lay flat on the floor and perform this movement by raising the upper body upwards slowly pause for 2 seconds at the top. Then slowly reverse the movement under control.

Chapter 10:

CALVES
DEVELOP SHAPELY CALVES

DEVELOP SHAPELY CALVES

10 DEVELOP SHAPELY CALVES

DEVELOP SHAPELY CALVES

Develop shapely calves

The calves add a finished look to the lower leg with a diamond shape. This muscle has three heads (muscle parts) the soleus, this is under the large lateral head and gives the calves a fully developed look viewed from the side and back.

The lateral and medial heads are on the outside and in the middle of the muscle. The gastrocnemius make up the majority of the calf muscle. However, the longer the gastroc, the larger the potential for enhanced calf muscle development. The stretch component adds strength, shape and muscle development in double quick time.

DEVELOP SHAPELY CALVES

10 DEVELOP SHAPELY CALVES

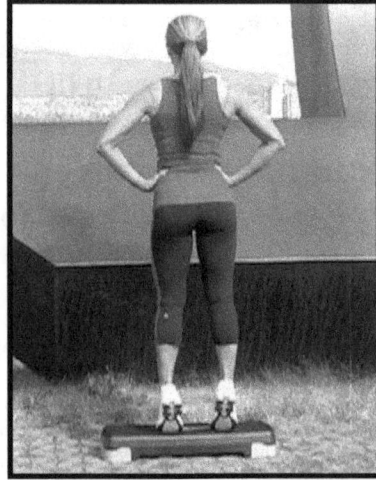

STANDING CALVE RAISES

Position yourself as shown but make sure the calves are well stretched. Start off as shown in the picture start position. Press straight up on the toes then lower. This is as awesome calve stretch exercise. Perform this exercise until the calves are well tired. This stimulates the entire calve.

Chapter 11:

ABDOMINALS
DEVELOP RIPPED ABS

DEVELOP RIPPED ABS

11 DEVELOP RIPPED ABS

The abdominal muscles are very important and reveal that the trainee has a lean physique. Plus, the role of the abdominal muscles is to protect the spine. A lean chiseled set of abdominal muscles shows the opposite sex that the owner has a sign of virility.

Once these muscles are well developed this keeps the waist line and belly flat. There are various muscle structures that complete the overall look, the entire length of the abdominal wall, plus the internal and external obliques.

The lower sections of the abdominal muscles play the largest role in protecting the spine and storing belly fat. This is the easiest place for body-fat to accumulate. Which makes training with self resistance the ideal exercise to attack those muscle fibers to the maximum.

DEVELOP RIPPED ABS

11 DEVELOP RIPPED ABS

DEVELOP RIPPED ABDOMINALS

As noted in the introduction the abdominal wall includes four muscles: Let's cover the entire length from the chest to pubis is called the rectus abdominis, people say abs for short. The abdominal wall should be worked in three angles of flexion. The lower sections of the abdominal muscles. The upper sections of the abdominal wall, and the obliques. Which are rotator muscles.

DEVELOP RIPPED ABS

11 DEVELOP RIPPED ABS

SIDE TO SIDE LATERAL RAISES

Normally people say I want to get rid of my love handles.
This abdominal exercise really isolates the oblique muscles.
These muscles support the spine by making the abdominal wall
more rigid. Start off as shown, spread the Iso-Bow apart maintaining the tension, Then lower the legs side to side.

DEVELOP RIPPED ABS

11 DEVELOP RIPPED ABS

REVERSE CRUNCHES

As shown above, place your hands under your butt slowly raise the legs upwards towards the chest or stomach. Pause for a 1 second count then slowly reverse the movement. This exercise stimulates the entire abdominal wall.

DEVELOP RIPPED ABS

11 DEVELOP RIPPED ABS

ABDOMINAL CRUNCHES

Lay on your back. Place the hands at your ear, tilt your head back, focus on the ceiling and crunch upward as shown.
DO NOT PULL ON THE HEAD.

Chapter 12:

POWER PUMP STANDARD PROGRAM

**PERFORM 30 FULL REPS. REP SPEED 3 SECONDS CONTRACTED
3 SECONDS RELEASE.
ALL PHASES ARE TO BE PERFORMED FOR 2 WEEKS DO NOT SKIP PHASES**

STANDARD PROGRAM PHASE ONE

12 PHASE ONE

MONDAY, WEDNESDAY, FRIDAY

Perform 30 reps at 3 sets each before moving to the next exercise. On the 30th rep perform a 10 second Isometric contraction at the middle of the exercise stroke. Perform each exercise using 50% of force.

STANDARD PROGRAM PHASE ONE

12 PHASE ONE

MONDAY, WEDNESDAY, FRIDAY
Routine continued.........

STANDARD PROGRAM PHASE ONE

12 PHASE ONE

MONDAY, WEDNESDAY, FRIDAY
Routine continued...........

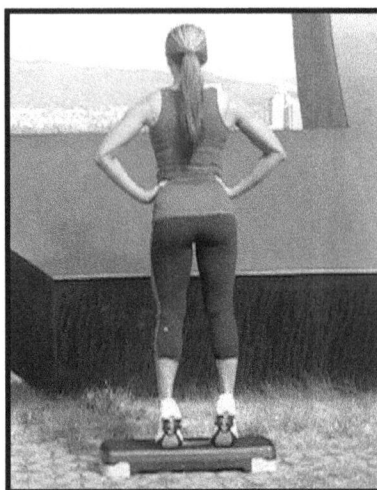

PHASE ONE MON, WED, FRI

STANDARD PROGRAM PHASE ONE

12 PHASE ONE

TUESDAY, THURSDAY, SATURDAY

Perform 30 reps at 3 sets each before moving to the next exercise. On the 30th rep perform a 10 second Isometric contraction at the middle of the exercise stroke. Perform each exercise using 50% of force.

STANDARD PROGRAM PHASE ONE

12 PHASE ONE

TUESDAY, THURSDAY, SATURDAY
Continued routine..........

STANDARD PROGRAM PHASE ONE

12 PHASE ONE

TUESDAY, THURSDAY, SATURDAY
Continued routine........

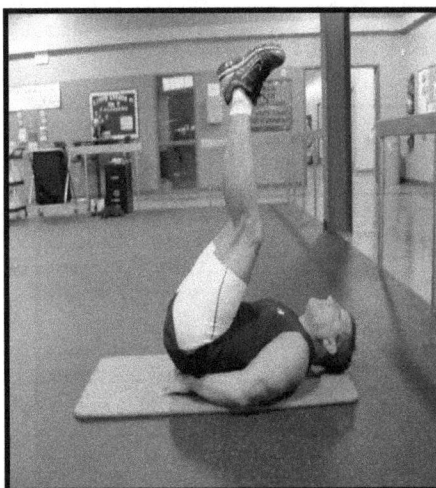

PHASE ONE TUES, THURS, SAT.

STANDARD PROGRAM PHASE TWO

13 PHASE TWO

MONDAY, WEDNESDAY, FRIDAY

Perform 10 reps at 3 sets each before moving to the next exercise. On the 10th rep perform a 20 second Isometric contraction at the middle of the exercise stroke. Perform each exercise using 50% of force.

Perform plan for 2 weeks

STANDARD PROGRAM PHASE TWO

13 PHASE TWO

MONDAY, WEDNESDAY, FRIDAY
ROUTINE CONTINUED........

PHASE TWO   MON, WED, FRI.

STANDARD PROGRAM PHASE TWO

13 PHASE TWO

TUESDAY, THURSDAY, SATURDAY

Perform 10 reps at 3 sets each before moving to the next exercise. On the 10th rep perform a 20 second Isometric contraction at the middle of the exercise stroke. Perform each exercise using 50% of force.

STANDARD PROGRAM PHASE TWO

13 PHASE TWO

TUESDAY, THURSDAY, SATURDAY

ROUTINE CONTINUED..........

PHASE TWO   TUES, THURS, SAT.

Chapter 14:

POWER PUMP
FIBER FUSION X2
REP SPEED 3 SECOND CONTRACTION
3 SECOND RELEASE 3 WEEKS

WEEK ONE: 15 REPS PER EXERCISE
WEEK TWO: 10 REPS PER EXERCISE
WEEK THREE: 7-9 REPS PER EXERCISE

FIBER FUSION X2

14 FIBER FUSION X2

HOW TO PERFORM THIS ROUTINE:
WEEK ONE:15 Reps per exercise
WEEK TWO:10 Reps per exercise
WEEK THREE:7-9 Reps per exercise
PERFORM 3 SETS EACH EXERCISE

DAY ONE

FIBER FUSION X2

14 FIBER FUSION X2

HOW TO PERFORM THIS ROUTINE:
WEEK ONE: 15 Reps per exercise
WEEK TWO: 10 Reps per exercise
WEEK THREE: 7-9 Reps per exercise
PERFORM 3 SETS EACH EXERCISE

DAY ONE continued..........

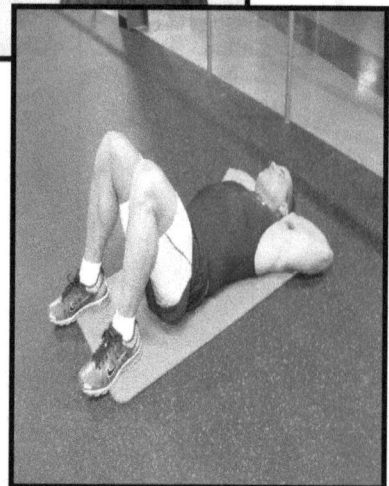

FIBER FUSION X2

14 FIBER FUSION X2

HOW TO PERFORM THIS ROUTINE:
WEEK ONE: 15 Reps per exercise
WEEK TWO: 10 Reps per exercise
WEEK THREE: 7-9 Reps per exercise
PERFORM 3 SETS EACH EXERCISE

DAY TWO

FIBER FUSION X2

14 FIBER FUSION X2

HOW TO PERFORM THIS ROUTINE:
WEEK ONE: 15 Reps per exercise
WEEK TWO: 10 Reps per exercise
WEEK THREE: 7-9 Reps per exercise
PERFORM 3 SETS EACH EXERCISE

DAY TWO continued............

FIBER FUSION X2

14 FIBER FUSION X2

HOW TO PERFORM THIS ROUTINE:
WEEK ONE:15 Reps per exercise
WEEK TWO:10 Reps per exercise
WEEK THREE:7-9 Reps per exercise
PERFORM 3 SETS EACH EXERCISE

DAY THREE

FIBER FUSION X2

14 FIBER FUSION X2

HOW TO PERFORM THIS ROUTINE:
WEEK ONE: 15 Reps per exercise
WEEK TWO: 10 Reps per exercise
WEEK THREE: 7-9 Reps per exercise
PERFORM 3 SETS EACH EXERCISE

DAY THREE continued.......

FIBER FUSION X2

14 FIBER FUSION X2

HOW TO PERFORM THIS ROUTINE:
WEEK ONE: 15 Reps per exercise
WEEK TWO: 10 Reps per exercise
WEEK THREE: 7-9 Reps per exercise
PERFORM 3 SETS EACH EXERCISE

DAY THREE continued.......

FIBER FUSION X2

14 FIBER FUSION X2

HOW TO PERFORM THIS ROUTINE:
WEEK ONE: 15 Reps per exercise
WEEK TWO: 10 Reps per exercise
WEEK THREE: 7-9 Reps per exercise
PERFORM 3 SETS EACH EXERCISE

DAY FOUR

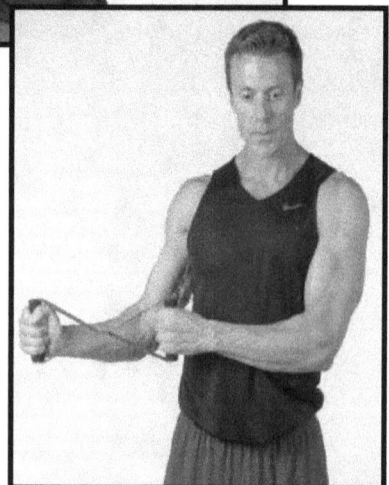

FIBER FUSION X2

14 FIBER FUSION X2

HOW TO PERFORM THIS ROUTINE:
WEEK ONE: 15 Reps per exercise
WEEK TWO: 10 Reps per exercise
WEEK THREE: 7-9 Reps per exercise
PERFORM 3 SETS EACH EXERCISE

DAY FOUR continued......

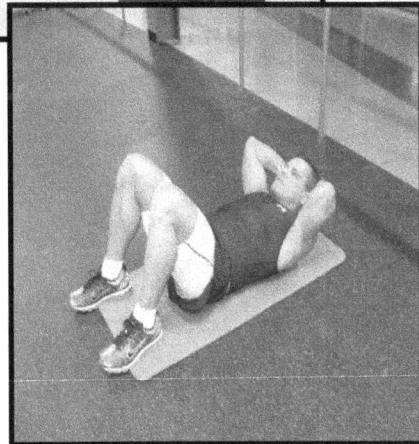

FIBER FUSION X2

14 FIBER FUSION X2

HOW TO PERFORM THIS ROUTINE:
WEEK ONE: 15 Reps per exercise
WEEK TWO: 10 Reps per exercise
WEEK THREE: 7-9 Reps per exercise
PERFORM 3 SETS EACH EXERCISE

DAY FIVE

FIBER FUSION X2

14 FIBER FUSION X2

HOW TO PERFORM THIS ROUTINE:
WEEK ONE:15 Reps per exercise
WEEK TWO:10 Reps per exercise
WEEK THREE:7-9 Reps per exercise
PERFORM 3 SETS EACH EXERCISE

DAY FIVE continued.....

THE POWER PUMP POWER SURGE PROGRAM PHASE ONE

THE POWER PUMP POWER SURGE PROGRAM

15 PHASE ONE

HOW TO PERFORM THIS ROUTINE:
PHASE ONE POWER PHASE

Perform 30 full reps, followed by 10 reps from the start to middle point of the exercise stroke. On the 10th rep perform a 5-7 second isometric contraction. One set per exercise. **REP SPEED 3 SECONDS CONTRACTED, 3 SECONDS RELEASE. Follow plan for 2 weeks.**

DAY ONE

THE POWER PUMP POWER SURGE PROGRAM

15 PHASE ONE

HOW TO PERFORM THIS ROUTINE:
PHASE ONE POWER PHASE

Perform 30 full reps, followed by 10 reps from the start to middle point of the exercise stroke. On the 10th rep perform a 5-7 second isometric contraction. One set per exercise. **REP SPEED 3 SECONDS CONTRACTED, 3 SECONDS RELEASE**

DAY ONE continued............

THE POWER PUMP POWER SURGE PROGRAM

15 PHASE ONE

HOW TO PERFORM THIS ROUTINE:
PHASE ONE POWER PHASE

Perform 30 full reps, followed by 10 reps from the start to middle point of the exercise stroke. On the 10th rep perform a 5-7 second isometric contraction. One set per exercise. **REP SPEED 3 SECONDS CONTRACTED, 3 SECONDS RELEASE**

DAY TWO

THE POWER PUMP POWER SURGE PROGRAM

15 PHASE ONE

HOW TO PERFORM THIS ROUTINE:
PHASE ONE POWER PHASE

Perform 30 full reps, followed by 10 reps from the start to middle point of the exercise stroke. On the 10th rep perform a 5-7 second isometric contraction. One set per exercise. **REP SPEED 3 SECONDS CONTRACTED, 3 SECONDS RELEASE**

DAY TWO continued.......

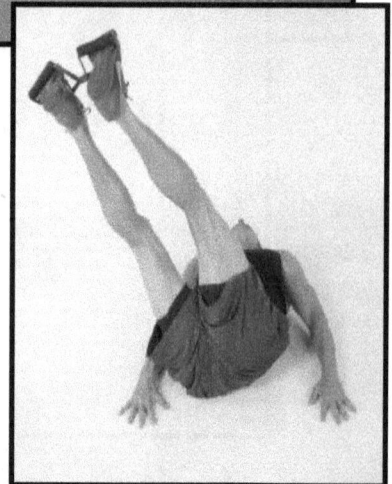

THE POWER PUMP POWER SURGE PROGRAM

15 PHASE ONE

HOW TO PERFORM THIS ROUTINE:
PHASE ONE POWER PHASE

Perform 30 full reps, followed by 10 reps from the start to middle point of the exercise stroke. On the 10th rep perform a 5-7 second isometric contraction. One set per exercise. **REP SPEED 3 SECONDS CONTRACTED, 3 SECONDS RELEASE**

DAY THREE

THE POWER PUMP POWER SURGE PROGRAM

15 PHASE ONE

HOW TO PERFORM THIS ROUTINE:
PHASE ONE POWER PHASE

Perform 30 full reps, followed by 10 reps from the start to middle point of the exercise stroke. On the 10th rep perform a 5-7 second isometric contraction. One set per exercise. **REP SPEED 3 SECONDS CONTRACTED, 3 SECONDS RELEASE**

DAY THREE continued..........

THE POWER PUMP POWER SURGE PROGRAM

15 PHASE ONE

HOW TO PERFORM THIS ROUTINE:
PHASE ONE POWER PHASE

Perform 30 full reps, followed by 10 reps from the start to middle point of the exercise stroke. On the 10th rep perform a 5-7 second isometric contraction. One set per exercise. **REP SPEED 3 SECONDS CONTRACTED, 3 SECONDS RELEASE**

DAY FOUR

THE POWER PUMP POWER SURGE PROGRAM

15 PHASE ONE

HOW TO PERFORM THIS ROUTINE:
PHASE ONE POWER PHASE

Perform 30 full reps, followed by 10 reps from the start to middle point of the exercise stroke. On the 10th rep perform a 5-7 second isometric contraction. One set per exercise. **REP SPEED 3 SECONDS CONTRACTED, 3 SECONDS RELEASE**

DAY FIVE

THE POWER PUMP POWER SURGE PROGRAM

15 PHASE ONE

HOW TO PERFORM THIS ROUTINE:
PHASE ONE POWER PHASE

Perform 30 full reps, followed by 10 reps from the start to middle point of the exercise stroke. On the 10th rep perform a 5-7 second isometric contraction. One set per exercise. **REP SPEED 3 SECONDS CONTRACTED, 3 SECONDS RELEASE**

DAY FIVE continued............

Chapter 15:

THE POWER PUMP POWER SURGE PROGRAM PHASE TWO

THE POWER PUMP POWER SURGE PROGRAM

15 PHASE TWO

HOW TO PERFORM THIS ROUTINE:
PHASE TWO

Contract within 2 seconds then reverse the movement for 4 seconds.
Perform 20 reps. On the 20th perform an isometric hold for 10 seconds.
Alternate day one and day two for 6 days per week. One set per exercise.
Perform this program for 2 weeks.

DAY ONE

THE POWER PUMP POWER SURGE PROGRAM

15 PHASE TWO

HOW TO PERFORM THIS ROUTINE:
PHASE TWO

Contract within 2 seconds then reverse the movement for 4 seconds. Perform 20 reps. On the 20th perform an isometric hold for 10 seconds. Alternate day one and day two for 6 days per week. One set per exercise. Perform this program for 2 weeks.

DAY ONE continued.........

THE POWER PUMP POWER SURGE PROGRAM

15 PHASE TWO

HOW TO PERFORM THIS ROUTINE:
PHASE TWO

Contract within 2 seconds then reverse the movement for 4 seconds.
Perform 20 reps. On the 20th perform an isometric hold for 10 seconds.
Alternate day one and day two for 6 days per week. One set per exercise.
Perform this program for 2 weeks.

DAY TWO

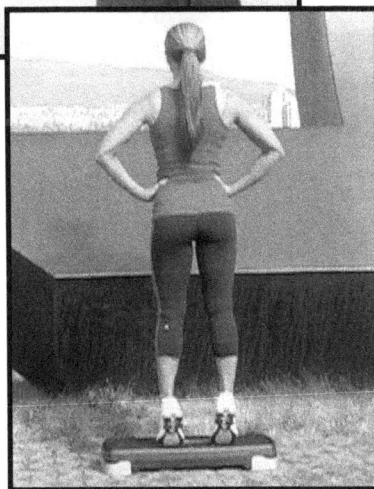

THE POWER PUMP POWER SURGE PROGRAM

15 PHASE TWO

HOW TO PERFORM THIS ROUTINE:
PHASE TWO

Contract within 2 seconds then reverse the movement for 4 seconds.
Perform 20 reps. On the 20th perform an isometric hold for 10 seconds.
Alternate day one and day two for 6 days per week. One set per exercise.
Perform this program for 2 weeks.

DAY TWO continued........

Chapter 15:

THE POWER PUMP POWER SURGE PROGRAM PHASE THREE

THE POWER PUMP POWER SURGE PROGRAM

15 PHASE THREE

HOW TO PERFORM THIS ROUTINE:
PHASE THREE

Perform 3-5 full reps —by contracting for 4 seconds and release 6 seconds. On the 5th rep perform 15 half reps, start to mid-point. Alternate day one and day two for 6 days per week. Perform 1-2 sets per exercise.
Perform plan for 2 weeks

DAY ONE

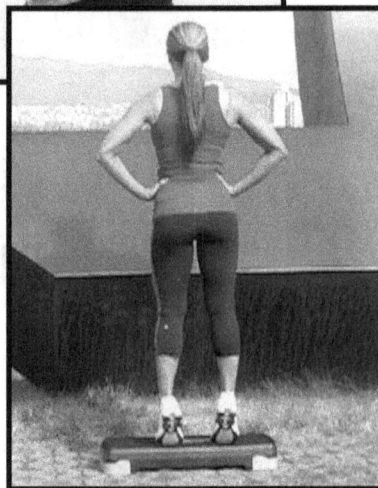

THE POWER PUMP POWER SURGE PROGRAM

15 PHASE THREE

HOW TO PERFORM THIS ROUTINE:
PHASE THREE

Perform 3-5 full reps —by contracting for 4 seconds and release 6 seconds. On the 5th rep perform 15 half reps, start to mid-point. Alternate day one and day two for 6 days per week. Perform 1-2 sets per exercise.

DAY ONE continued...........

THE POWER PUMP POWER SURGE PROGRAM

15 PHASE THREE

HOW TO PERFORM THIS ROUTINE:
PHASE THREE

Perform 3-5 full reps —by contracting for 4 seconds and release 6 seconds. On the 5th rep perform 15 half reps, start to mid-point. Alternate day one and day two for 6 days per week. Perform 1-2 sets per exercise.

DAY TWO

THE POWER PUMP POWER SURGE PROGRAM

15 PHASE THREE

HOW TO PERFORM THIS ROUTINE:
PHASE THREE

Perform 3-5 full reps —by contracting for 4 seconds and release 6 seconds. On the 5th rep perform 15 half reps, start to mid-point. Alternate day one and day two for 6 days per week. Perform 1-2 sets per exercise.

DAY TWO continued...........

We are looking forward to hearing from you on your progress. Please drop us an email skippymarl@icloud. com